THE BASIC KETO CHICKEN RECIPES

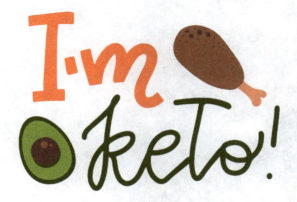

The Perfect Collection of Delicious &

Keto Chicken Recipes and More

Royal Keto

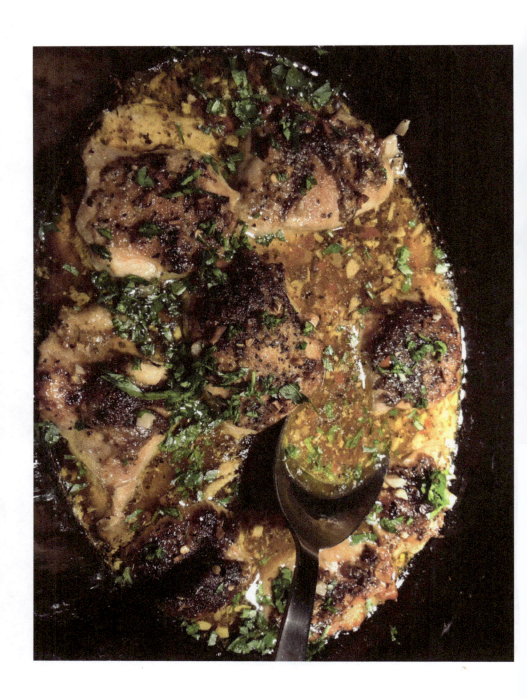

© Copyright 2021 by KetoRoyal- All rights reserved. The following Book is reproduced below with the goal of providing information that is as accurate and reliable as possible. Regardless, purchasing this Book can be seen as consent to the fact that both the publisher and the author of this book are in no way experts on the topics discussed within and that any recommendations or suggestions that are made herein are for entertainment purposes only. Professionals should be consulted as needed prior to undertaking any of the action endorsed herein. This declaration is deemed fair and valid by both the American Bar Association and the Committee of Publishers Association and is legally binding throughout the United States. Furthermore, the transmission, duplication, or reproduction of any of the following work including specific information will be considered an illegal act irrespective of if it is done electronically or in print. This extends to creating a secondary or tertiary copy of the work or a recorded copy and is only allowed with the express written consent from the Publisher. All additional right reserved. The information in the following pages is broadly considered a truthful and accurate account of facts and as such, any inattention, use, or misuse of the information in question by the reader will render any resulting actions solely under their purview. There are no scenarios in which the publisher or the original author of this work can be in any fashion deemed liable for any hardship or damages that may befall them after undertaking information described herein. Additionally, the information in the following pages is intended only for informational purposes and should thus be thought of as universal. As befitting its nature, it is presented without assurance regarding its prolonged validity or interim quality. Trademarks that are mentioned are done without written consent and can in no way be considered an endorsement from the trademark holder.

KETO CHICKEN RECIPES AND MORE 1

- Chicken Liver Stew 8
- Balsamic Chicken 10
- Low - Carb Butternut Chicken 13
- Greek Chicken Breast 15
- Filet Mignon & Mushrooms Sauce 17
- Beef Kabobs 20
- Keto Steaks and Scallops 22
- Beef Medallions Mix 24
- Balsamic Beef 26
- Pork Chops and Roasted Peppers 28
- Pork Chops and Green Beans 30
- Pork Chops and Sage Sauce 32
- Ham and Veggie Air Fried Mix 34
- Simple Green Goddess Dressing 36
- Keto Béchamel Sauce 38
- Avocado Mayo Medley 40
- Amazing Garlic Aioli 42
- Lovely Herbed Cream Cheese 44
- Good Looking Butter Mayo 46
- Spicy Wasabi Mayonnaise 48
- The Cowboy Sauce 50
- Creative Lamb Chops 52
- Crazy Lamb Salad 54
- Healthy Slow-Cooker Lamb Leg 57
- Spicy Paprika Lamb Chops 59
- Lamb Riblets & Mini Pesto 61
- Terrific Jalapeno Bacon Bombs 63
- Beautiful Mushroom Pork Chops 66
- Lemon & Garlic Pork Platter 68
- The Herbal Buttery Pork Chops 71
- Italian Pork Chops 73
- Cheesy Pork Chops 75
- Delicious Caramelized Pork Chops 77
- Simple Pork Stuffed Bell Peppers 79
- Parmesan Pork Steak 81
- Slow Cooked Cranberry & Pork Roast 83
- Satisfyingly Spicy Pork Chops 85
- Oven Baked Slow Baked Pork Shoulder 87
- Onion & Bacon Pork Chops 89
- Beef & Egg Early Muffin 91
- Italian Parmesan Baked Chicken 93
- The Almond Breaded Chicken Goodness 95

- Brown Butter Duck Breast 97
- Healthy Chicken Cream Salad 99
- Salsa Chicken 101
- Clean Chicken & Mushroom Stew 103
- Hearty Keto Chicken & Egg Soup 105
- Healthy Lamb Stew 107

Chicken Liver Stew

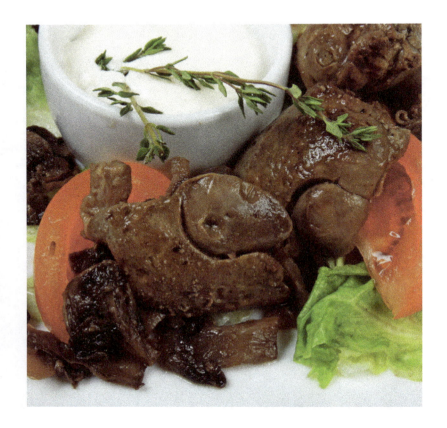

Serving: 2

Prep Time: 10 minutes

Ingredients

- 10 ounces chicken livers
- 1 ounce onion, chopped
- 2 ounces sour cream
- 1 tablespoon olive oil

- Salt to taste

How To

1. Take a pan and place it over medium heat
2. Add oil and let it heat up
3. Add onions and fry until just browned
4. Add livers and season with salt
5. Cook until livers are half cooked
6. Transfer the mix to a stew pot
7. Add sour cream and cook for 20 minutes
8. Serve and enjoy!

Balsamic Chicken

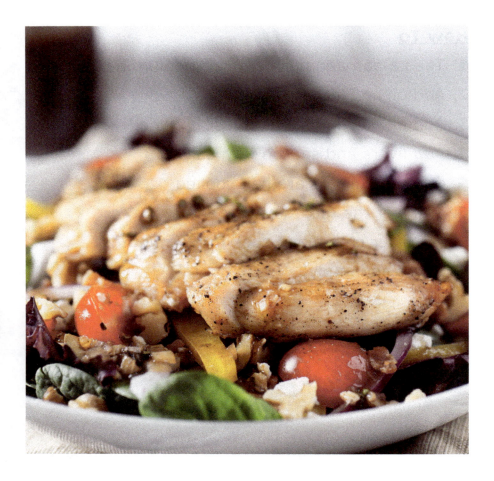

Serving: 6

<u>Ingredients</u>

- 6 chicken breast halves, skinless and boneless
- 1 teaspoon garlic salt
- 1 teaspoon dried oregano

- 1 teaspoon dried rosemary
- ½ teaspoon dried thyme
- Ground black pepper
- 2 tablespoons olive oil
- 1 onion, thinly sliced
- 14 and ½ ounces tomatoes, diced
- ½ cup balsamic vinegar
- 1 teaspoon dried basil

How To

1. Season both sides of your chicken breasts thoroughly with pepper and garlic salt
2. Take a skillet and place it over medium heat
3. Add some oil and cook your seasoned chicken for 3-4 minutes per side until the breasts are nicely browned
4. Add some onion and cook for another 3-4 minutes until the onions are browned
5. Pour the diced up tomatoes and balsamic vinegar over your chicken and season with some rosemary, basil, thyme and rosemary
6. Simmer the chicken for about 15 minutes until they are no longer pink

7. Take an instant read thermometer and check if the internal temperature gives a reading of 165 degree Fahrenheit

8. If yes, then you are good to go!

Low - Carb Butternut Chicken

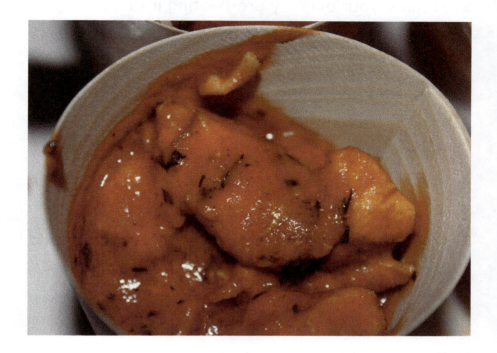

Serving: 4

Ingredients

- 2-3 cups butternut squash, cubed
- Extra virgin olive oil
- Fresh chopped sage
- ½ pound Nitrate free bacon
- 6 chicken thighs, boneless and skinless
- Salt and pepper as needed

How To

1. Prepare your oven by pre-heating it to 425 degree F
2. Take a large skillet and place it over medium-high heat, add bacon and fry until crispy
3. Take a bacon and place it on the side, crumbled the bacon
4. Add cubed butternut squash in the bacon grease and Saute, season with salt and pepper
5. Once the squash is tender, remove skillet and transfer to plate
6. Add coconut oil to the skillet and add chicken thigh, cook for 10 minutes
7. Season with salt and pepper
8. Remove skillet from stove and transfer to oven
9. Bake for 12-15 minutes, top with crumbled bacon and sage

Enjoy!

Greek Chicken Breast

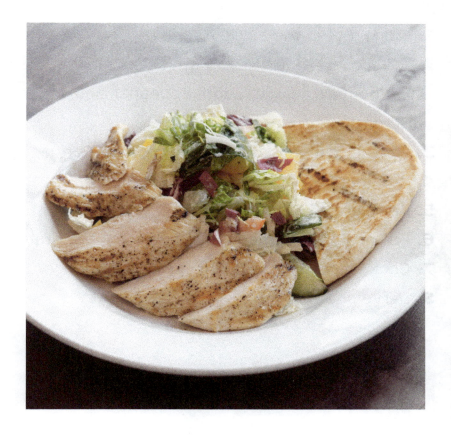

Serving: 4

Ingredients

- 2 teaspoons garlic, crushed
- 1 and ½ teaspoons black pepper
- 1/3 teaspoon paprika
- 4 chicken breast halves, skinless and boneless
- 1 cup extra virgin olive oil

- 1 lemon, juiced

How To

1. Cut 3 slits in the chicken breast
2. Take a small bowl and whisk in olive oil, salt, lemon juice, garlic, paprika, pepper and whisk for 30 seconds
3. Place chicken in large bowl and pour marinade
4. Rub marinade all over using your hand
5. Refrigerate overnight
6. Pre-heat grill to medium heat and oil the grate
7. Cook chicken in grill until center is no longer pink
8. Serve and enjoy!

Filet Mignon & Mushrooms Sauce

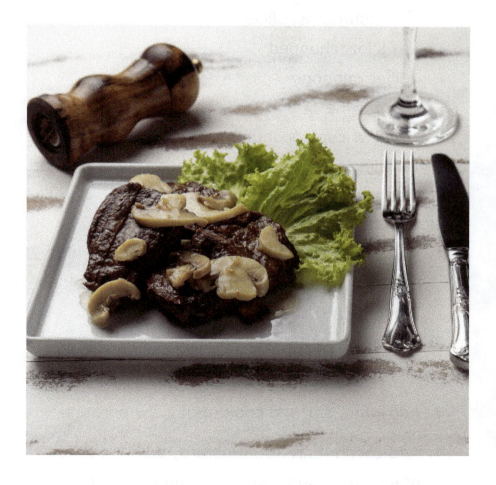

Preparation time: 10 minutes

Cooking time: 25 minutes

Servings: 4

Ingredients:

- 2 garlic cloves, minced
- 2 tablespoons olive oil
- ¼ cup Dijon mustard
- 12 mushrooms, sliced
- 1 shallot, chopped
- 4 fillet mignons
- ¼ cup wine
- 1 and ¼ cup coconut cream
- 2 tablespoons parsley, chopped
- Salt and black pepper to the taste

Directions:

1. Heat up a pan with the oil over medium high heat, add garlic and shallots, stir and cook for 3 minutes.
2. Add mushrooms, stir and cook for 4 minutes more.
3. Add wine, stir and cook until it evaporates.
4. Add coconut cream, mustard, parsley, a pinch of salt and black pepper to the taste, stir, cook for 6 minutes more and take off heat.

5. Season fillets with salt and pepper, put them in your air fryer and cook at 360 degrees F for 10 minutes.
6. Divide fillets on plates and serve with the mushroom sauce on top.

Enjoy!

Beef Kabobs

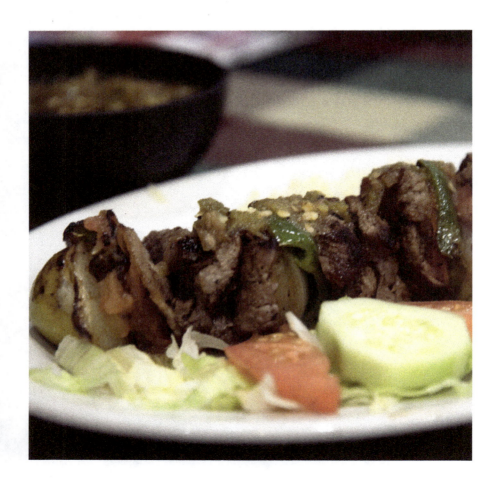

Preparation time: 10 minutes

Cooking time: 10 minutes

Servings: 4

Ingredients:

- ¼ cup olive oil
- ¼ cup salsa

- Salt and black pepper to the taste
- 2 red bell peppers, chopped
- 2 pounds sirloin steak, cut into medium pieces
- 1 red onion, chopped
- 1 zucchini, sliced
- Juice form 1 lime
- 2 tablespoons chili powder
- 2 tablespoon hot sauce
- ½ tablespoons cumin, ground

Directions:

1. In a bowl, mix salsa with lime juice, oil, hot sauce, chili powder, cumin, salt and black pepper and whisk well.

2. Divide meat bell peppers, zucchini and onion on skewers, brush kabobs with the salsa mix you made earlier, put them in your preheated air fryer and cook them for 10 minutes at 370 degrees F flipping kabobs halfway.

3. Divide among plates and serve with a side salad.

Enjoy!

Keto Steaks and Scallops

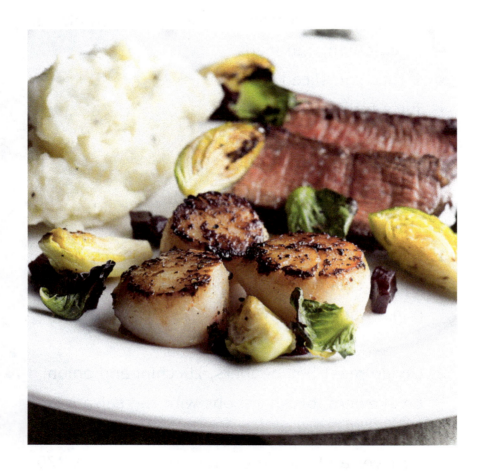

Preparation time: 10 minutes
Cooking time: 14 minutes
Servings: 2
Ingredients:
- 10 sea scallops

- 2 beef steaks
- 4 garlic cloves, minced
- 1 shallot, chopped
- 2 tablespoons lemon juice
- 2 tablespoons parsley, chopped
- 2 tablespoons basil, chopped
- 1 teaspoon lemon zest
- ¼ cup butter
- ¼ cup veggie stock
- Salt and black pepper to the taste

Directions:

1. Season steaks with salt and pepper, put them in your air fryer, cook at 360 degrees F for 10 minutes and transfer to a pan that fits the fryer.
2. Add shallot, garlic, butter, stock, basil, lemon juice, parsley, lemon zest and scallops, toss everything gently and cook at 360 degrees F for 4 minutes more.
3. Divide steaks and scallops on plates and serve.

Enjoy!

Beef Medallions Mix

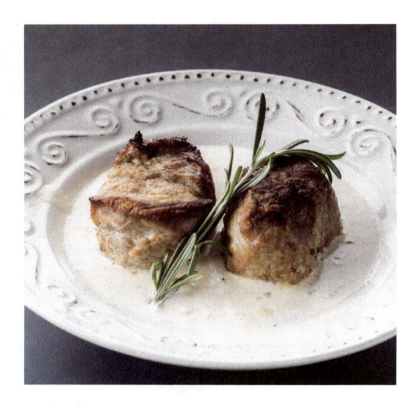

Preparation time: 2 hours

Cooking time: 10 minutes

Servings: 4

Ingredients:

- 2 teaspoons chili powder
- 1 cup tomatoes, crushed
- 4 beef medallions
- 2 teaspoons onion powder

- 2 tablespoons soy sauce
- Salt and black pepper to the taste
- 1 tablespoons hot pepper
- 2 tablespoons lime juice

Directions:
1. In a bowl, mix tomatoes with hot pepper, soy sauce, chili powder, onion powder, a pinch of salt, black pepper and lime juice and whisk well.
2. Arrange beef medallions in a dish, pour sauce over them, toss and leave them aside for 2 hours.
3. Discard tomato marinade, put beef in your preheated air fryer and cook at 360 degrees F for 10 minutes.
4. Divide steaks on plates and serve with a side salad.

Enjoy!

Balsamic Beef

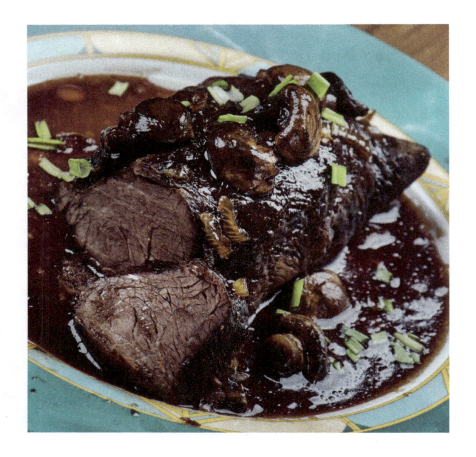

Preparation time: 10 minutes

Cooking time: 1 hour

Servings: 6

Ingredients:

- 1 medium beef roast
- 1 tablespoon Worcestershire sauce

- ½ cup balsamic vinegar
- 1 cup beef stock
- 1 tablespoons honey
- 1 tablespoon soy sauce
- 4 garlic cloves, minced

Directions:
1. In a heat proof dish that fits your air fryer, mix roast with roast with Worcestershire sauce, vinegar, stock, honey, soy sauce and garlic, toss well,
2. Introduce in your air fryer and cook at 370 degrees F for 1 hour.

3. Slice roast, divide among plates, drizzle the sauce all over and serve. Enjoy!

Pork Chops and Roasted Peppers

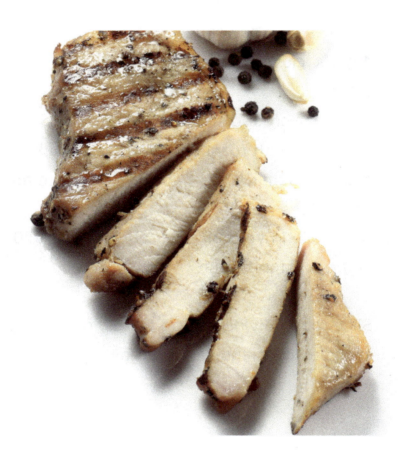

Preparation time: 10 minutes

Cooking time: 16 minutes

Servings: 4

Ingredients:

- 3 tablespoons olive oil

- 3 tablespoons lemon juice
- 1 tablespoon smoked paprika
- 2 tablespoons thyme, chopped
- 3 garlic cloves, minced
- 4 pork chops, bone in
- Salta and black pepper to the taste
- 2 roasted bell peppers, chopped

Directions:

1. In a pan that fits your air fryer, mix pork chops with oil, lemon juice, smoked paprika, thyme, garlic, bell peppers, salt and pepper, toss well,
2. Introduce in your air fryer and cook at 400 degrees F for 16 minutes.
3. Divide pork chops and peppers mix on plates and serve right away. Enjoy!

Pork Chops and Green Beans

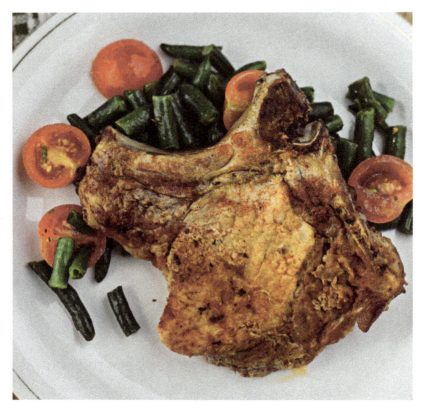

Preparation time: 10 minutes

Cooking time: 15 minutes

Servings: 4

Ingredients:

- 4 pork chops, bone in
- 2 tablespoons olive oil
- 1 tablespoon sage, chopped
- Salt and black pepper to the taste

- 16 ounces green beans
- 3 garlic cloves, minced
- 2 tablespoons parsley, chopped

Directions:
1. In a pan that fits your air fryer, mix pork chops with olive oil, sage, salt, pepper, green beans, garlic and parsley, toss,
2. Introduce in your air fryer and cook at 360 degrees F for 15 minutes.
3. Divide everything on plates and serve.

Enjoy!

Nutrition: calories 261, fat 7, fiber 9, carbs 14, protein 20

Pork Chops and Sage Sauce

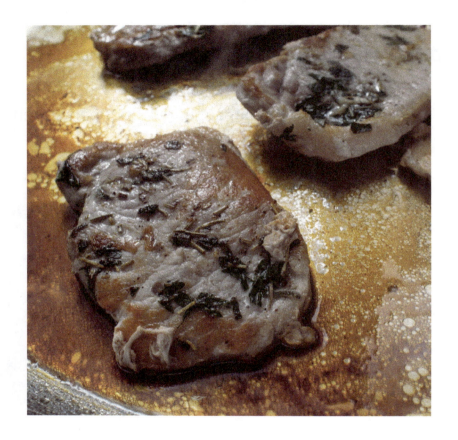

Preparation time: 10 minutes

Cooking time: 15 minutes

Servings: 2

Ingredients:

- 2 pork chops
- Salt and black pepper to the taste
- 1 tablespoon olive oil

- 2 tablespoons butter
- 1 shallot, sliced
- 1 handful sage, chopped
- 1 teaspoon lemon juice

Directions:

1. Season pork chops with salt and pepper, rub with the oil, put in your air fryer and cook at 370 degrees F for 10 minutes, flipping them halfway.
2. Meanwhile, heat up a pan with the butter over medium heat, add shallot, stir and cook for 2 minutes.
3. Add sage and lemon juice, stir well, cook for a few more minutes and take off heat.
4. Divide pork chops on plates, drizzle sage sauce all over and serve.

Enjoy!

Ham and Veggie Air Fried Mix

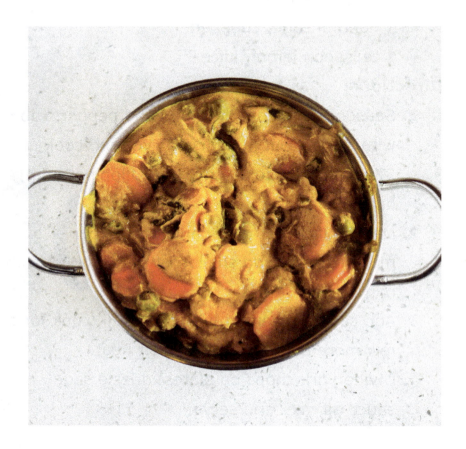

Preparation time: 10 minutes
Cooking time: 20 minutes
 Servings: 6
Ingredients:
- ¼ cup butter
- ¼ cup flour

- 3 cups milk
- ½ teaspoon thyme, dried
- 2 cups ham, chopped
- 6 ounces sweet peas
- 4 ounces mushrooms, halved
- 1 cup baby carrots

Directions:

1. Heat up a large pan that fits your air fryer with the butter over medium heat, melt it, add flour and whisk well.
2. Add milk and, well again and take off heat.
3. Add thyme, ham, peas, mushrooms and baby carrots, toss,
4. Put in your air fryer and cook at 360 degrees F for 20 minutes.
5. Divide everything on plates and serve.

Enjoy!

Simple Green Goddess Dressing

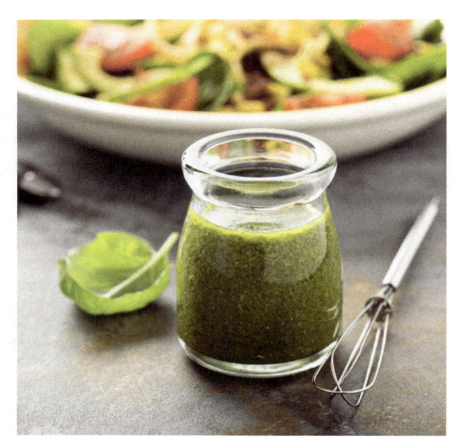

Serving: 2

Prep Time: 5 minutes

Ingredients

- 2 tablespoons buttermilk
- ¼ cup Greek yogurt
- 1 teaspoon apple cider vinegar
- 1 garlic clove, minced

- 1 tablespoon olive oil
- 1 tablespoon fresh parsley leaves

How To

1. Take a food processor and add butter, milk, yogurt, vinegar, apple cider, garlic, olive oil, parsley and blend well until combined

2. Pour into sealed glass container and chill for 30 minutes

3. Use as needed!

Keto Béchamel Sauce

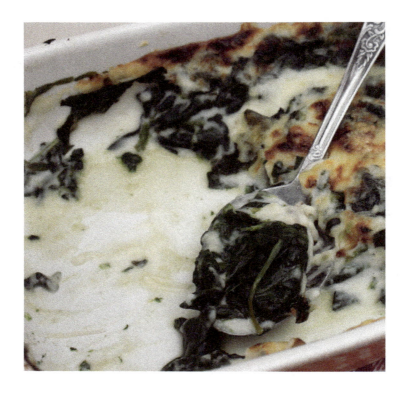

Serving: 6

Prep Time: 5 minutes

Cook Time: 5-7 minutes

Ingredients

- ½ teaspoon salt
- ¼ teaspoon ground black pepper
- ¼ teaspoon nutmeg
- 1 and ¾ cups heavy whip cream

- 7 ounces cream cheese

How To

1. Add listed ingredients to a non-stick saucepan and bring to a boil, making sure to keep stirring it continuously

2. Lower heat to low and let it simmer for a few minutes until it reaches your desired consistency

3. Once done, season with salt and pepper and use as needed!

Avocado Mayo Medley

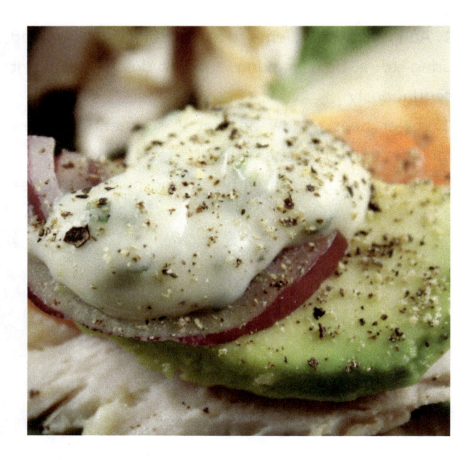

Serving: 4

Prep Time: 5 minutes

Ingredients

- 2 tablespoons fresh cilantro
- Pinch of salt
- ¼ cup olive oil

- 1 medium avocado, cut into chunks
- ½ teaspoon ground cayenne pepper

How To

1. Take a food processor and add avocado, cayenne pepper, lime juice, salt and cilantro

2. Mix until smooth

3. Slowly incorporate olive oil, add 1 tablespoon at a time and keep processing in between additions

4. Store and use as needed!

Enjoy!

Amazing Garlic Aioli

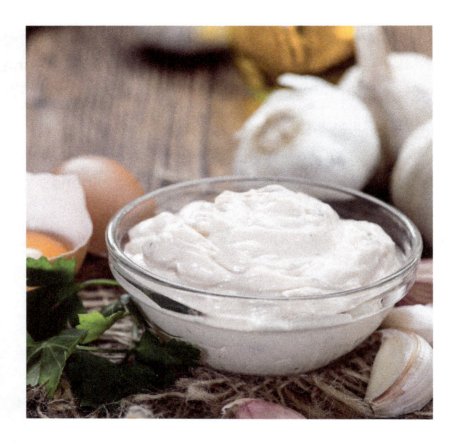

Serving: 4

Prep Time: 5 minutes

Ingredients

- ½ cup mayonnaise
- Salt and pepper to taste
- 2 garlic cloves, minced

- Juice of 1 lemon
- 1 tablespoon fresh-flat leaf Italian parsley, chopped
- 1 teaspoon chives, chopped

How To

1. Add mayo, garlic, parsley, lemon juice, chives and season with salt and pepper

2. Blend until combined well

3. Pour into refrigerator and chill for 30 minutes

4. Serve and enjoy using Keto Friendly bread!

Lovely Herbed Cream Cheese

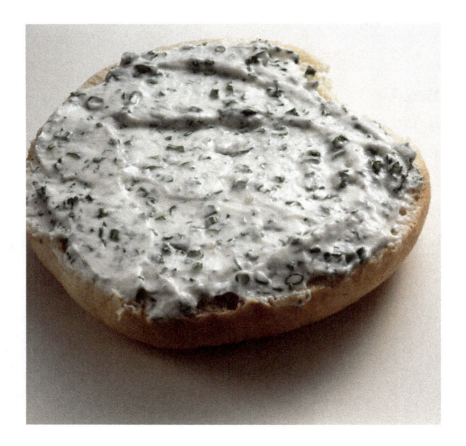

Serving: 4

Prep Time: 15 minutes

Ingredients

- ½ cup fresh parsley, chopped
- 1 garlic clove
- ½ lemon, zest

- Salt and pepper to taste
- 8 ounce cream cheese
- 2 teaspoons olive oil

How To

1. Take a bowl and mix everything

2. Let it sit in fridge for 15 minutes

3. Serve and enjoy!

Good Looking Butter Mayo

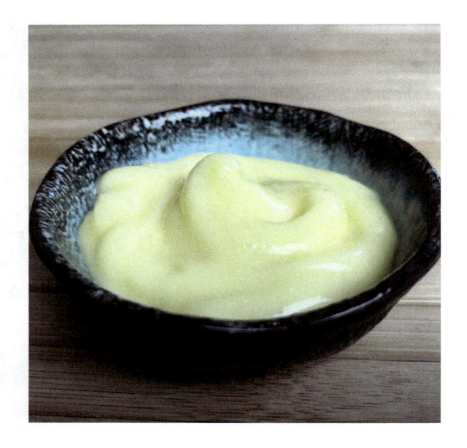

Serving: 4

Prep Time: 15 minutes

Cook Time: 1 minute

Ingredients

- 1 tablespoon Dijon mustard
- 1 teaspoon lemon juice

- ¼ teaspoon salt
- 1 pinch ground black pepper
- 5 and 1/3 ounces butter
- 1 egg yolk

How To

1. Take a saucepan and melt butter

2. Pour into a small pitcher and let it cool

3. Take a bowl and mix in egg yolks and mustard

4. Pour butter into a thin stream and keep beating using hand mixer

5. Leave sediment at bottom

6. Keep beating until mixture thickens

7. Add lemon juice and season with salt and pepper

8. Use as needed!

Spicy Wasabi Mayonnaise

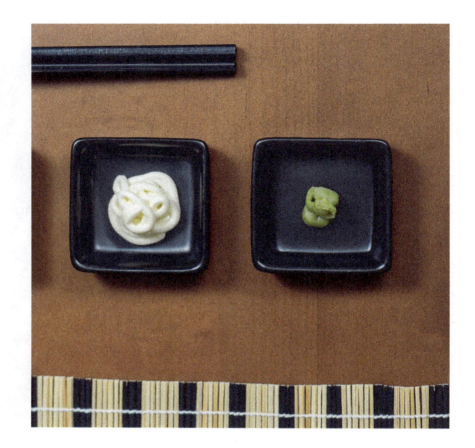

Serving: 4

Prep Time: 15 minutes

Ingredients

- ½ tablespoon wasabi paste
- 1 cup mayonnaise

How To

1. Take a bowl and mix wasabi paste and mayonnaise
2. Mix well
3. Let it chill and use as needed

The Cowboy Sauce

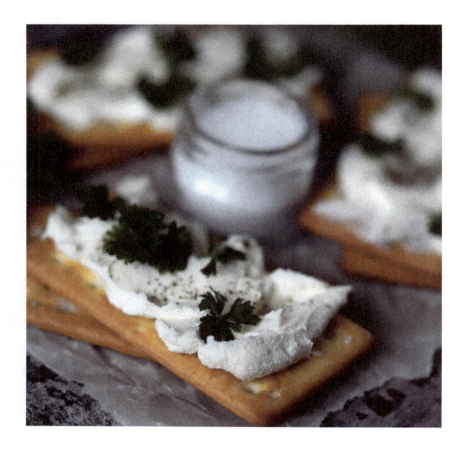

Serving: 4

Prep Time: 5 minutes

Cook Time: 5 minutes

Ingredients

- 1 scallion, chopped
- 1 tablespoon fresh chives, chopped

- 1 tablespoon fresh horseradish, grated
- 1 teaspoon dried thyme
- 7 ounces butter
- 2 garlic cloves, chopped
- 1 teaspoon paprika powder
- ½ teaspoon salt
- 1 pinch cayenne pepper

How To

1. Melt butter over medium heat in a saucepan

2. Add remaining ingredients

3. Whisk vigorously while simmer until sauce thickens

4. Serve and enjoy!

Creative Lamb Chops

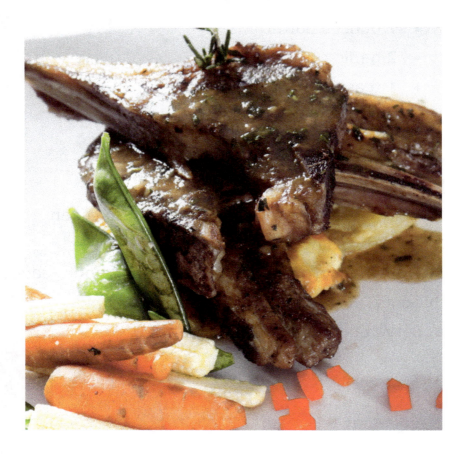

Serving: 3

Prep Time: 35 minutes

Cook Time: 5 minutes

<u>Ingredients</u>

- 8 lamb rib chops
- 1 tablespoon garlic, minced

- ¼ cup olive oil
- ¼ cup mint, fresh and chopped
- 1 tablespoon rosemary, fresh and chopped

How To

1. Add rosemary, garlic, mint, olive oil into a bowl and mix well

2. Keep a tablespoon of the mixture on the side for later use

3. Toss lamb chops into the marinade, letting them marinate for 30 minutes

4. Take a cast iron skillet and place it over medium-high heat

5. Add lamb and cook for 2 minutes per side for medium rare

6. Let the lamb rest for a few minutes and drizzle remaining marinade

7. Serve and enjoy!

Crazy Lamb Salad

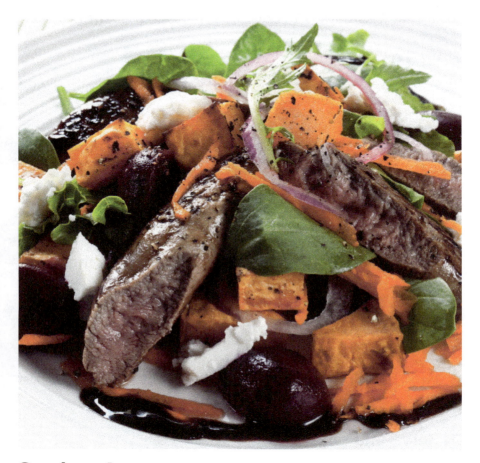

Serving: 4
Prep Time: 10 minutes
Cook Time: 35 minutes
<u>Ingredients</u>

- 1 tablespoon olive oil
- 1 teaspoon cumin

- Pinch of dried thyme
- 3 pounds leg of lamb, bone removed, leg butterflied
- Salt and pepper to taste
- 2 garlic cloves, peeled and minced

For Salad
- 2 cups spinach
- 1 and ½ tablespoons lemon juice
- ¼ cup olive oil
- 4 ounces feta cheese, crumbled
- ½ cup pecans
- 1 cup fresh mint, chopped

How To

1. Rub lamb with salt and pepper, 1 tablespoon oil, thyme, cumin, minced garlic

2. Pre-heat your grill to medium-high h and transfer lamb

3. Cook for 40 minutes, making sure to flip it once

4. Take a lined baking sheet and spread pecans

5. Toast in oven for 10 minutes at 350 degree F

6. Transfer grilled lamb to cutting board and let it cool

7. Slice

8. Take a salad bowl and add spinach, 1 cup mint, feta cheese, ¼ cup olive oil, lemon juice, toasted pecans, salt, pepper and toss well
9. Add lamb slices on top
10. Serve and enjoy!

Healthy Slow-Cooker Lamb Leg

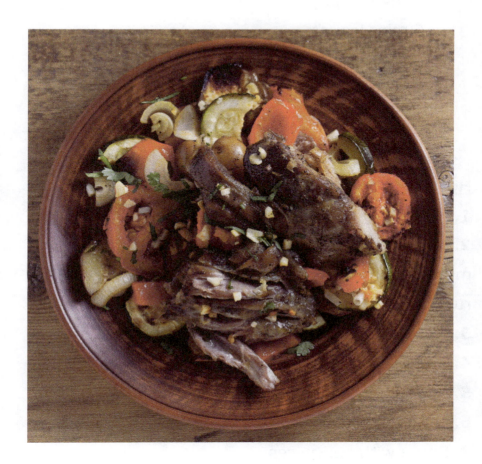

Serving: 6

Prep Time: 10 minutes

Cook Time: 8 hours

Ingredients

- 2 pounds lamb leg
- Salt and pepper to taste

- ¼ cup olive oil
- 4 thyme sprigs
- 6 mint leaves
- 1 teaspoon garlic, minced
- 1 tablespoon vanilla bean extract
- 2 tablespoons mustard
- Pinch of dried rosemary

How To

1. Add oil to your Slow Cooker
2. Add lamb, salt, pepper, vanilla bean extract, mustard, rosemary, garlic to your Slow Cooker and rub the mixture well
3. Place lid and cook on LOW for 7 hours
4. Add mint and thyme
5. Cook for 1 hour more
6. Let it cool and slice
7. Serve with pan juices
8. Enjoy!

Spicy Paprika Lamb Chops

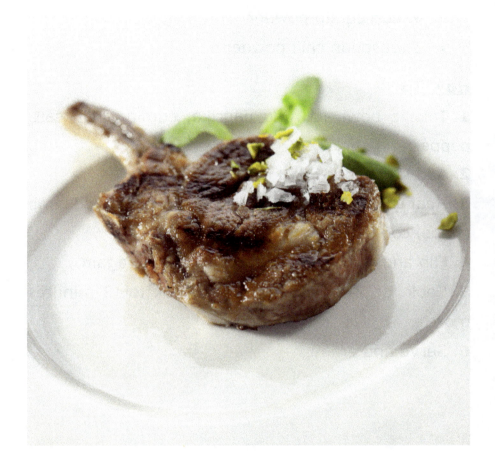

Serving: 4

Prep Time: 10 minutes

Cook Time: 15 minutes

<u>Ingredients</u>

- Salt and pepper to taste

- 3 tablespoons paprika
- 2 lamb racks, cut into chops
- ¾ cup cumin powder
- 1 teaspoon chili powder

How To

1. Take a bowl and add paprika, cumin, chili, salt, pepper and stir

2. Add lamb chops and rub the mixture

3. Heat grill over medium-temperature and add lamb chops, cook for 5 minutes

4. Flip and cook for 5 minutes more, flip again

5. Cook for 2 minutes, flip and cook for 2 minutes more

6. Serve and enjoy!

Lamb Riblets & Mini Pesto

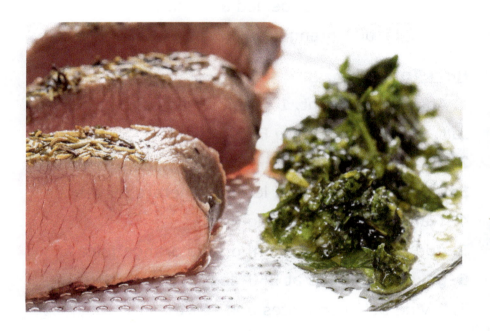

Serving: 4

Prep Time: 60 minutes

Cook Time: 120 minutes

<u>Ingredients</u>

- 1 and ½ onions, peeled and chopped
- 1/3 cup pistachios
- 1 teaspoon lemon zest
- 1 cup parsley
- 1 cup mint
- 5 tablespoons avocado oil

- Salt, to taste
- 2 pounds lamb riblets
- 5 garlic cloves, peeled and minced
- Juice of 1 orange

How To

1. Add parsley, mint, 1 onion, pistachios, lemon zest, salt, and avocado oil to Food processor

2. Rub lamb with mix

3. Transfer to bowl and let it refrigerate for 1 hour

4. Transfer lamb to baking dish

5. Add garlic and ½ onion, drizzle orange juice

6. Bake for 2 hours at 250-degree F

7. Divide between plates and serve

8. Enjoy!

Terrific Jalapeno Bacon Bombs

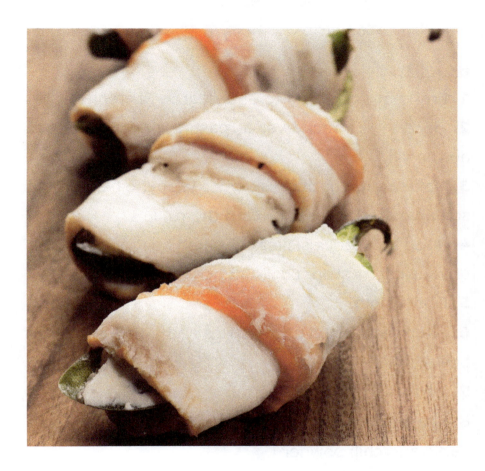

Serving: 2

Prep Time: 15 minutes

Cook Time: 10 minutes

Ingredients

- 6 ounce of full fat cream cheese
- 2 teaspoon of garlic powder

- 1 teaspoon of chili powder
- 12 large jalapeno peppers
- 16 bacon strips

How To

1. Pre-heat your oven to 350-degree Fahrenheit

2. Place a wire rack over a roasting pan and keep it on the side

3. Make a slit lengthways across jalapeno pepper and scrape out the seeds, discard them

4. Place a nonstick skillet over high heat and add half of your bacon strip, cook until crispy

5. Drain them

6. Chop the cooked bacon strips and transfer to large bowl

7. Add cream cheese and mix

8. Season the cream cheese and bacon mix with garlic and chili powder

9. Mix well

10. Stuff the mix into the jalapeno peppers with and wrap raw bacon strip all around

11. Arrange the stuffed wrapped jalapeno on prepare wire rack

12. Roast for 10 minutes

13. Transfer to cooling rack and serve! Enjoy!

Beautiful Mushroom Pork Chops

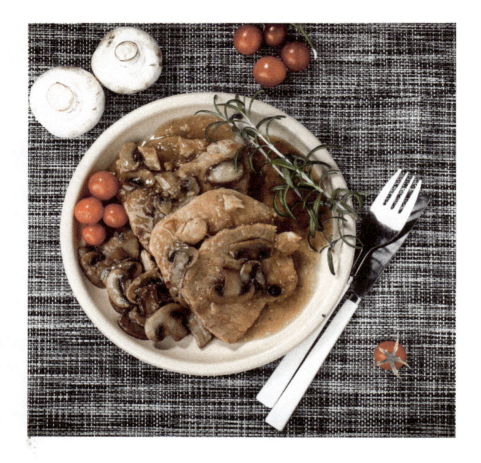

Serving: 3

Ingredients

- 8 ounces mushrooms, sliced
- 1 tablespoon balsamic vinegar
- ½ cup coconut oil
- 1 teaspoon garlic

- 1 onion, peeled and chopped
- 1 cup Keto-Friendly Mayonnaise
- 3 pork chops, boneless
- 1 teaspoon ground nutmeg

How To

1. Take a pan and place it over medium heat

2. Add oil and let it heat up

3. Add mushrooms, onions and stir

4. Cook for 4 minutes

5. Add pork chops, season with nutmeg, garlic powder and brown both sides

6. Transfer the pan in oven and bake for 30 minutes at 350-degree F

7. Transfer pork chops to plates and keep it warm

8. Take a pan and place it over medium-heat

9. Add vinegar, mayonnaise over mushroom mix and stir or a few minutes

10. Drizzle sauce over pork chops

11. Enjoy!

Lemon & Garlic Pork Platter

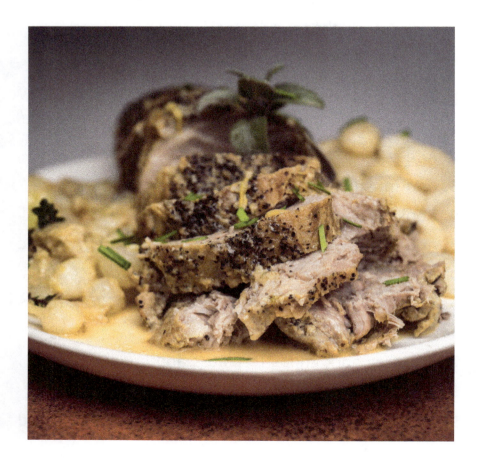

Serving: 4

Prep Time: 10 minutes

Cook Time: 30 minutes

Ingredients

- 1 cup chicken stock
- Salt and pepper to taste

- Pinch of lemon pepper
- 3 tablespoons coconut oil
- 6 garlic cloves, peeled and minced
- 2 tablespoons fresh parsley, chopped
- 8 ounces mushrooms, chopped
- 1 lemon, sliced 3 tablespoons butter
- 4 pork steak, bone-in

How To

1. Take a pan and place it over medium medium-high heat

2. Add 2 tablespoons butter and 2 tablespoon oil, let it heat up

3. Add pork steaks and season with salt and pepper

4. Cook until browned on both sides

5. Transfer to plate

6. Return pan to medium heat and add remaining butter, oil and half of stock

7. Stir well and cook for 1 minute

8. Add mushrooms, garlic, stir cook for 4 minutes

9. Add lemon slices , remaining stock, slat, pepper and lemon pepper

10. Stir cook for 5 minutes

11. Return steaks to pan and cook for 10 minutes

12. Divide steak and sauce between serving platters
13. Enjoy!

The Herbal Buttery Pork Chops

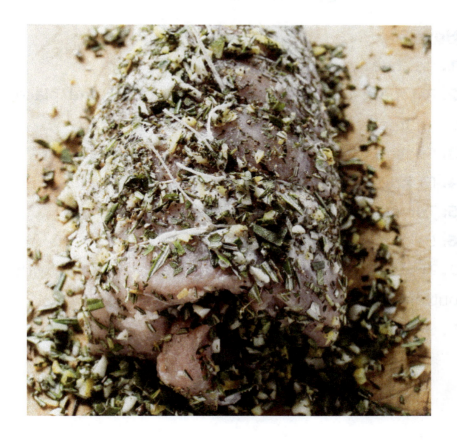

Serving: 3

Prep Time: 5 minutes

Cook Time: 25 minutes

Ingredients

- Salt and pepper to taste
- 1 tablespoon dried Italian seasoning
- 1 tablespoon olive oil

- 1 tablespoon butter, divided
- 2 boneless pork chops

How To

1. Pre-heat your oven to 350-degree F

2. Pat pork chops dry with paper towel and place them in a baking dish

3. Season with salt, pepper and Italian seasoning

4. Drizzle olive oil over pork chops

5. Top each chop with ½ tablespoon butter

6. Bake for 25 minutes

7. Transfer pork chops on two plates and top with butter juice

8. Serve and enjoy!

Italian Pork Chops

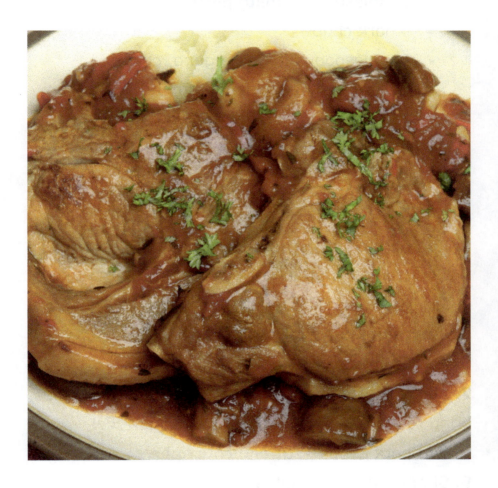

Serving: 4

Prep Time: 10 minutes

Cook Time: 37 minutes

Ingredients

- 1 tablespoon canola oil

- 15 ounces canned tomatoes, diced
- 1 tablespoon tomato paste
- 4 pork chops
- 1 tablespoons fresh oregano, chopped
- 2 garlic cloves, peeled and minced
- Salt and pepper to taste
- ¼ cup tomato juice

How To

1. Heat up pan with oil over medium-high heat

2. Add pork chops, season with salt and pepper

3. Cook for 3 minutes

4. Flip and cook for 3 minutes more

5. Return the pan to medium heat

6. Add garlic and stir cook for 10 seconds

7. Add tomato juice, tomato paste and tomatoes, bring to a boil and lower heat to medium-low

8. Add pork chops , stir and cover pan

9. Simmer for 30 minutes

10. Transfer chops to platter and add oregano to pan, stir cook for 2 minutes

11. Pour over pork chops

12. Serve and enjoy!

Cheesy Pork Chops

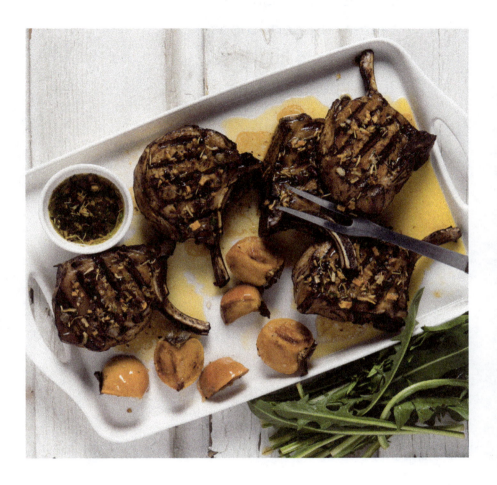

Serving: 4

Prep Time: 10 minutes

Cook Time: 25 minutes

Ingredients

- 1 whole egg

- Bacon grease for frying
- 3 ounces parmesan cheese
- 7 center cut, pork chops
- ½ cup almond flour
- Salt and pepper to taste

<u>How To</u>

1. Pre-heat your oven to 400-degree F

2. Take a bowl and mix in cheese, flour and seasoning

3. Take another bowl and mix in egg

4. Dip pork chops in eggs, followed by a dip in the flour /cheese mix

5. Fry in oil for 1-2 minutes each side (on medium heat)

6. Transfer to a baking dish and bake in oven until golden brown

7. Enjoy!

Delicious Caramelized Pork Chops

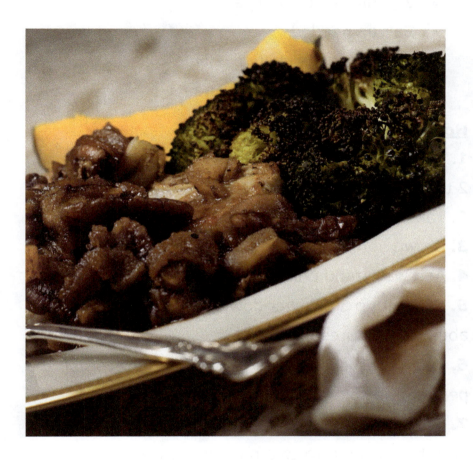

Serving: 4

Prep Time: 5 minutes

Cook Time: 30 minutes

Ingredients

- 4 pounds chuck roast

- 4 ounces green chili, chopped
- ½ teaspoon ground cumin
- 2 garlic cloves, minced
- Salt as needed
- 2 tablespoons chili powder
- ½ teaspoon dried oregano

How To

1. Rub up your chop with 1 teaspoon of pepper and 2 teaspoon of seasoning salt

2. Take a skillet and heat some oil over medium heat

3. Brown your pork chops on each sides

4. Add water and onions to the pan

5. Cover it up and lower down the heat, simmer it for about 20 minutes

6. Turn your chops over and add the rest of the pepper and salt

7. Cover it up and cook until the water evaporates and the onions turn to a medium brown texture

8. Remove the chops from your pan and serve with some onions on top!

Simple Pork Stuffed Bell Peppers

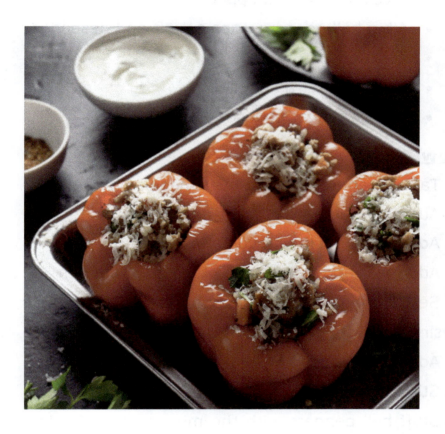

Serving: 4

Prep Time: 10 minutes

Cook Time: 26 minutes

Ingredients

- 1 teaspoon Cajun spice
- 1 pound pork, ground

- 1 tablespoons tomato paste
- 6 garlic cloves, minced
- 1 yellow onion, chopped
- 4 big bell peppers, tops cut off and deseeded
- Pinch of salt
- Black pepper as needed
- 1 cup cheddar cheese

How To

1. Take a pan and place it over medium-high heat

2. Add oil and let the oil heat up

3. Add garlic, onion and cook for 4 minutes

4. Add meat and gently stir cook for 10 minutes

5. Season with salt and pepper according to your desire

6. Add Cajun seasoning and tomato paste

7. Stir cook for 3 minutes more

8. Stuff bell peppers with the mix and transfer to a pre-heated grill, top with cheese

9. Grill for 3 minutes (each side)

10. Divide between plates and serve

11. Enjoy!

Parmesan Pork Steak

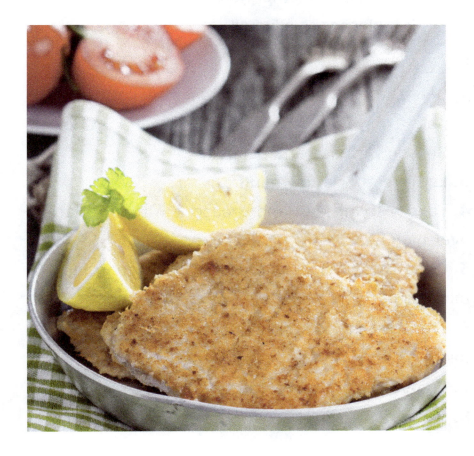

Serving: 4

Prep Time: 10 minutes

Cook Time: 15 minutes

Ingredients

- ½ pound pork steak
- Salt and pepper to taste

- 1 ounce parmesan, grated/melted
- 1 tablespoon lemon juice
- 2 tablespoons olive oil

How To

1. Beat the pork steak with kitchen mallet to flatten it a bit

2. Season with salt and pepper

3. Let it rest for a few minutes

4. Take a frying pan and grease it with oil, place it over high heat

5. Once the oil is hot, add steak and cook for 7-8 minutes per side

6. Transfer cooked steak on a plate and drizzle lemon juice

7. Cover with grated parmesan/melted parmesan

8. Serve and enjoy!

Slow Cooked Cranberry & Pork Roast

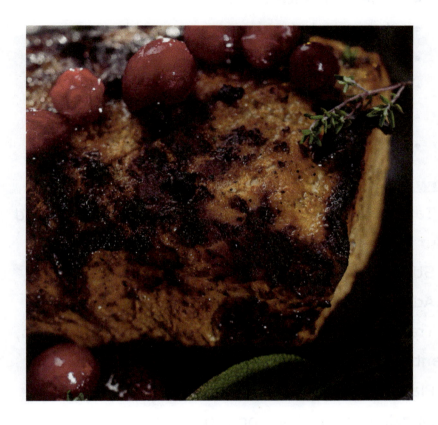

Serving: 4

Prep Time: 10 minutes

Cook Time: 8 hours

Ingredients

- 1 tablespoon coconut flour
- Salt and pepper to taste

- 1 and ½ pound pork loin
- Pinch of dry mustard
- ½ lemon, sliced
- ¼ cup water
- ½ teaspoon ginger
- 2 tablespoons stevia
- ½ cup cranberries
- 2 garlic cloves, peeled and minced

How To

1. Take a owl and add ginger, mustard, pepper and flour

2. Stir well

3. Add roast and toss well to coat it

4. Transfer meat to a Slow Cooker and add stevia, cranberries, garlic, water, lemon slices

5. Place lid and cook on LOW for 8 hours

6. Drizzle the pan juice on top and serve!

Nutrition (Per Serving)

- Calories: 430
- Fat: 23g
- Carbohydrates: 3g
- Protein: 45g

Satisfyingly Spicy Pork Chops

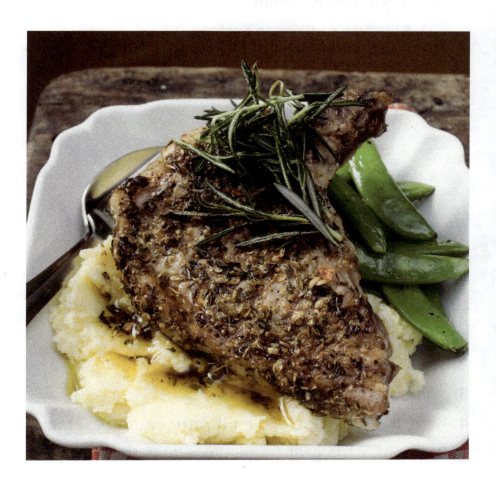

Serving: 4

Prep Time: 4 hours 10 minutes

Cook Time: 15 minutes

Ingredients

- 1 tablespoon chili powder

- 1 teaspoon ground cinnamon
- 2 teaspoons cumin
- Salt and pepper to taste
- ½ teaspoon hot pepper sauce
- Mango, sliced
- ¼ cup lime juice
- 4 pork rib chops
- 1 tablespoon coconut oil, melted
- 2 garlic cloves, peeled and minced

How To

1. Take a bowl and mix in lime juice, oil, garlic, cumin, cinnamon, chili powder, salt, pepper, hot pepper sauce

2. Whisk well

3. Add pork chops and toss

4. Keep it on the side and let it refrigerate for 4 hours

5. Pre-heat your grill to medium and transfer pork chops to pre-heated grill

6. Grill for 7 minutes, flip and cook for 7 minutes more

7. Divide between serving platters and serve with mango slices

8. Enjoy!

Oven Baked Slow Baked Pork Shoulder

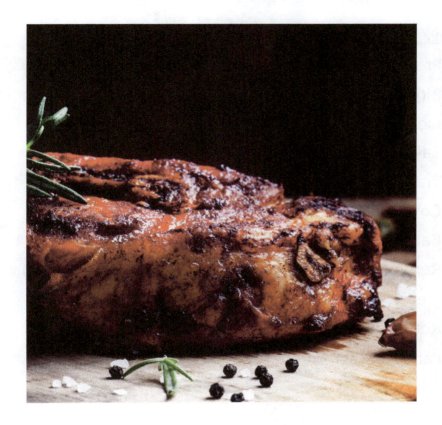

Serving: 4

Prep Time: 10 minutes

Cook Time: 9-10 hours 20 minutes

Ingredients

- 1 teaspoon garlic powder
- 1 teaspoon onion powder

- Salt and pepper to taste
- 4 pounds pork shoulder
- 2 teaspoons oregano

How To

1. Pre-heat your oven to 250 degree F

2. Rinse meat and wash well, rub the meat with seasoning

3. Take a roasting pan and cover with aluminum foil

4. Transfer meat to the pan

5. Cover with another foil and transfer to oven

6. Bake for 9-10 hours

7. Remove meat, increase oven temperature to 500 degree F

8. Return meat and bake for 15-20 minutes more

9. Let it cool, slice and enjoy!

Onion & Bacon Pork Chops

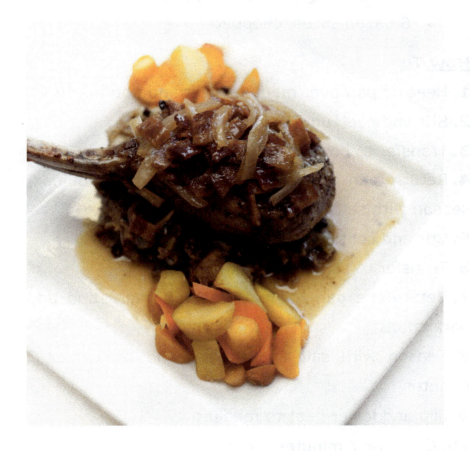

Serving: 4

Prep Time: 10 minutes

Cook Time: 45 minutes

Ingredients

- ½ cup chicken stock
- Salt and pepper to taste

- 4 pork chops
- 2 onions, peeled and chopped
- 6 bacon slices, chopped

How To

1. Heat up pan over medium-heat and add bacon
2. Stir and cook until crispy
3. Transfer to bowl
4. Return pan to medium heat and add onions, season with salt and pepper
5. Stir and cook for 15 minutes
6. Transfer to same bowl with bacon
7. Return the pan to heat (medium-high) and add pork chops
8. Season with salt and pepper and brown for 3 minutes
9. Flip and lower heat to medium
10. Cook for 7 minutes more
11. Add stock and stir cook for 2 minutes
12. Return the bacon and onions to the pan and stir cook for 1 minute
13. Serve and enjoy!

Nutrition (Per Serving)

- Calories: 325

Beef & Egg Early Muffin

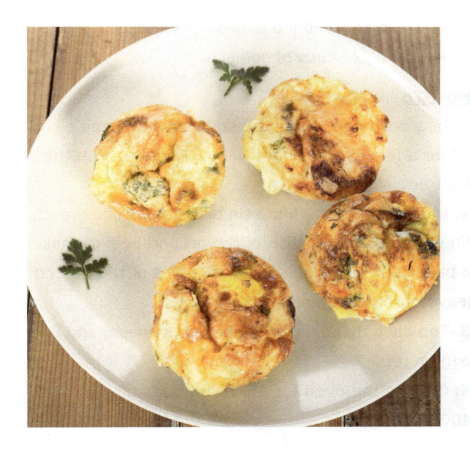

Serving: 12

Prep Time: 10 minutes

Cook Time: 15 minutes

<u>Ingredients</u>

- 2 lbs of ground beef (20% fat/80% lean meat ratio)

- 1 tbsp of mixed herbs
- 12 eggs
- 1 cup of shredded cheddar cheese
- 2 and 1/2 cups of spinach

How To

1. In a deep pan, saute the spinach with some olive oil for a few minutes until wilted. Remove from the heat and set aside.

2. In a 12-piece muffin, a tin dish begins lining each tin with around 1-2 tbsp of the ground beef to make a base cup. You should cover all sides of the tin and leave room for the spinach and eggs.

3. Top each meat cup with spinach, cheese, and one egg on top.

4. Cook in the oven for 15-18 minutes at 400F/200C

Italian Parmesan Baked Chic.

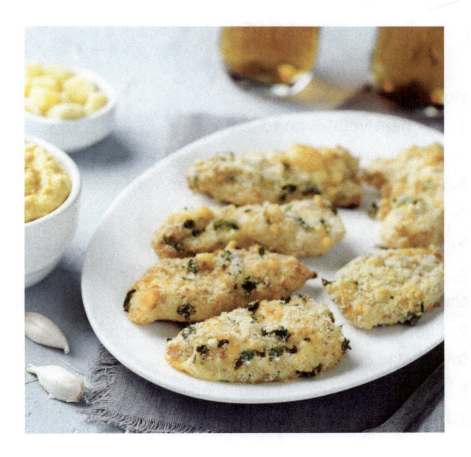

Serving: 2

Ingredients

- 2 tablespoons ghee
- ¼ cup parmesan cheese, grated
- 1 tablespoon dried Italian seasoning
- ¼ cup crushed pork rinds

- 2 boneless chicken breasts, skinless
- Pink salt
- Freshly ground black pepper
- ½ cup mayonnaise

<u>How To</u>

1. Pre-heat your oven to 425 degree F
2. Take a large baking dish and coat with ghee
3. Pat chicken breasts dry and wrap with towel
4. Season with salt and pepper
5. Place in baking dish
6. Take a small bowl and add mayonnaise, parmesan cheese, Italian seasoning
7. Slather mayo mix evenly over chicken breast
8. Sprinkle crushed pork rinds on top
9. Bake for 20 minutes until topping is browned
10. Serve and enjoy!

The Almond Breaded Chicken Goodness

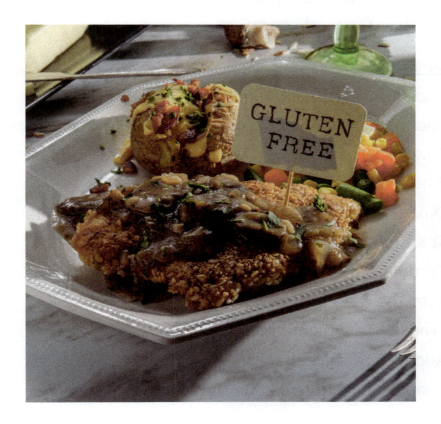

Serving: 3

Prep Time: 15 minutes

Cook Time: 15 minutes

<u>Ingredients</u>

- 1 and ½ cups seasoned almond meal
- 2 tablespoons coconut oil

- Lemon pepper, to taste
- 2 large chicken breast, boneless and skinless
- 1/3 cup lemon juice
- Parsley for decoration

How To

1. Slice chicken breast in half

2. Pound out each half until ¼ inch thick

3. Take a pan and place it over medium heat, add oil and heat it up

4. Dip each chicken breast slice into lemon juice and let it sit for 2 minutes

5. Turnover and the let the other side sit for 2 minutes as well

6. Transfer to almond meal and coat both sides

7. Add coated chicken to the oil and fry for 4 minutes per side, making sure to sprinkle lemon pepper liberally

8. Transfer to a paper lined sheet and repeat until all chicken are fried

9. Garnish with parsley and enjoy!

Brown Butter Duck Breast

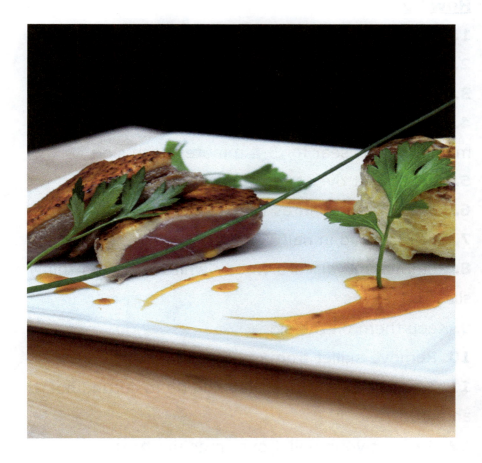

Serving: 3

<u>Ingredients</u>

- 1 head radicchio, 4 ounces, core removed
- ¼ cup unsalted butter
- 6 fresh sage leaves, sliced
- 1 whole 6 ounces duck breast, skin on

- Salt and pepper to taste

How To

1. Pre-heat your oven to 400 degree F
2. Pat duck breast dry with paper towel
3. Season with salt and pepper
4. Place duck breast in skillet and place it over medium heat, sear for 3-4 minutes each side
5. Turn breast over and transfer skillet to oven
6. Roast for 10 minutes (uncovered)
7. Cut radicchio in half
8. Remove and discard woody white core and thinly slice the leaves
9. Keep them on the side
10. Remove skillet from oven
11. Transfer duck breast, fat side up to cutting board and let it rest
12. Re-heat your skillet over medium heat
13. Add Unsalted butter, sage and cook for 3-4 minutes
14. Cut duck into 6 equal slices
15. Divide radicchio between 2 plates, top with slices of duck breast and drizzle browned butter and sage
16. Enjoy!

Healthy Chicken Cream Salad

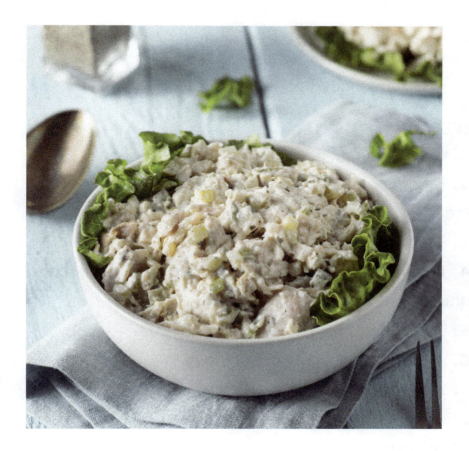

Serving: 3

Prep Time: 5 minutes

Cook Time: 50 minutes

Ingredients

- 3 ounces celery
- 2 ounce green pepper, chopped

- ½ ounce green onion, chopped
- 2 chicken breasts
- 1 and ½ cups heavy cream
- ½ cup Keto-Friendly mayo
- 3 hard-boiled eggs, chopped

How To

1. Pre-heat your oven to 350 degree F

2. Take a baking sheet and place chicken, cover with cream

3. Bake for 30-40 minutes

4. Take a bowl and mix in chopped celery, peppers, onions

5. Shred the baked chicken

6. Peel and chop hard boiled eggs

7. Take large salad bowl and mix in eggs, veggies and chicken

8. Toss well and serve

9. Enjoy!

Salsa Chicken

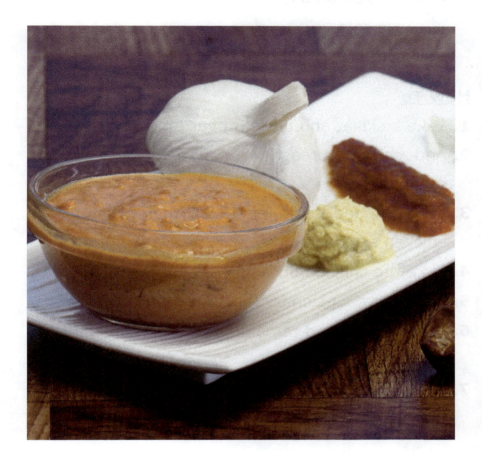

Serving: 4

Prep Time: 4 minutes

Cook Time: 14 minutes

Ingredients

- 1 cup plain Greek Yogurt
- ½ a cup of cheddar cheese, cubed

- 2 chicken breast
- 1 cup salsa
- 1 taco seasoning mix

How To

1. Take a skillet and place it over medium heat
2. Add chicken breast, ½ cup of salsa and taco seasoning
3. Mix well and cook for 12-15 minutes until the chicken are done
4. Take the chicken out and cube them
5. Place the cubes on toothpick and top with cheddar
6. Place yogurt and remaining salsa in cups and use as dips
7. Enjoy!

Clean Chicken & Mushroom Stew

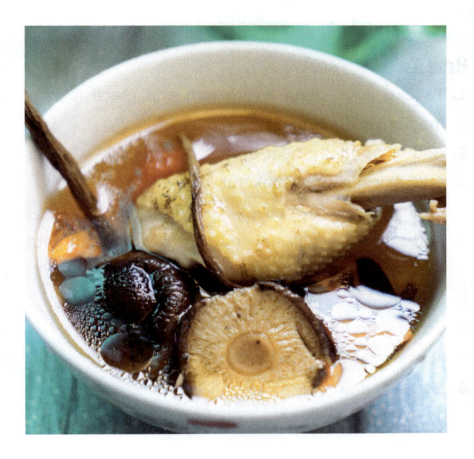

Serving: 4

<u>Ingredients</u>

- 4 chicken breast halves, cut into bite sized pieces
- 1 pound mushrooms, sliced (5-6 cups)
- 1 bunch spring onion, chopped

- 4 tablespoons olive oil
- 1 teaspoon thyme
- Salt and pepper as needed

How To

1. Take a large deep frying pan and place it over medium-high heat
2. Add oil and let it heat up
3. Add chicken and cook for 4-5 minutes per side until slightly browned
4. Add spring onions and mushrooms, season with salt and pepper according to your taste
5. Stir
6. Cover with lid and bring the mix to a boil
7. Lower heat and simmer for 25 minutes
8. Serve and Enjoy!

Hearty Keto Chicken & Egg Soup

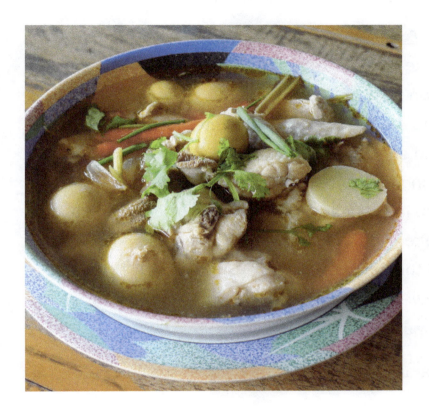

Serving: 2

Prep Time: 5 minutes

Cook Time: 10 minutes

<u>Ingredients</u>

- 1 and ½ cup chicken broth
- 2 whole eggs
- 1 teaspoon chili garlic paste

- 1 tablespoon bacon grease
- ½ a cube, chicken bouillon

How To

1. Take a stove top pan and place it over medium-high heat
2. Add chicken broth, bouillon cube, bacon grease and stir
3. Bring the mix to a boil
4. Mix in chili garlic paste
5. Take a bowl and whisk in eggs, add whisked egg to the pan
6. Lower down heat and gently simmer for a few minutes

Serve and enjoy!

Healthy Lamb Stew

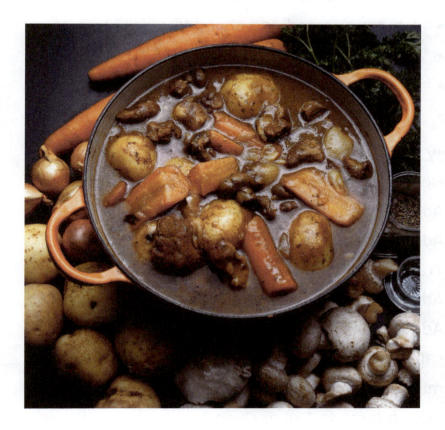

Serving: 4

Ingredients

- 1 cup white wine
- Salt and pepper to taste
- 2 rosemary sprigs
- 1 teaspoon fresh thyme, chopped
- 1 onion, peeled and chopped

- 3 carrots, peeled and chopped
- 2 pounds lamb, cubed
- 1 tomato, cored and chopped
- 1 garlic clove, peeled and minced
- 2 tablespoons butter
- 1 cup beef stock

How To

1. Heat up Dutch oven over medium-high heat
2. Add oil and let it heat up
3. Add lamb, salt, pepper and brown all sides
4. Transfer to plate
5. Add onion to Dutch oven and cook for 2 minutes
6. Add carrots, tomato, garlic, butter stick, wine, salt, pepper, rosemary, thyem and stir for a few minutes
7. Return lamb to Dutch Oven and cook for4 hours
8. Discard rosemary sprits
9. Add more salt, pepper and stir
10. Divide between bowls
11. Serve and enjoy!